SEATED YOGA FOR SENIORS

Gentle Fitness for Life Over 60

NATHAN TYLER

Table of contents

Introduction

Aging gracefully is not about avoiding the effects of time; it's about embracing each stage of life with strength, vitality, and peace of mind. For seniors, staying active plays a crucial role in maintaining both physical and mental well-being. However, traditional fitness routines may feel daunting, especially for those with mobility challenges or chronic conditions. This is where chair yoga becomes a game-changer.

Chair yoga offers a gentle yet effective way to stay active, increase flexibility, and nurture inner calm, all while being accessible to everyone, regardless of fitness level. By blending the time-honored traditions of yoga with the support of a chair, seniors can enjoy the transformative benefits of movement, mindfulness, and relaxation in a way that feels safe and enjoyable.

In this introduction, we'll explore the benefits of chair yoga for seniors, how it promotes graceful aging, and the essentials needed to embark on this empowering journey.

The Benefits of Chair Yoga for Seniors

Chair yoga is much more than a modified exercise routine—it's a holistic practice that nurtures the mind, body, and soul. Here are some of the key benefits:

1. Improved Flexibility

As we age, muscles and joints naturally lose some of their flexibility. Chair yoga involves gentle stretches that can help seniors regain and maintain a greater range of motion, reducing stiffness and enhancing daily activities like reaching, bending, or walking.

2. Enhanced Strength and Balance

Chair yoga includes poses that help strengthen muscles and improve balance, reducing the risk of falls—a common concern for seniors. Even seated postures engage the core and lower body, promoting stability and coordination.

3. Better Posture

Years of sitting and reduced physical activity can lead to poor posture, causing back and neck discomfort. Chair yoga strengthens the spine and encourages better alignment, relieving pain and promoting a more confident stance.

4. Stress and Anxiety Relief

Breathing techniques and mindfulness are integral to chair yoga. These practices help lower cortisol levels (the stress hormone), reduce anxiety, and create a sense of calm, which is particularly beneficial for seniors navigating life changes.

5. Improved Circulation and Joint Health

The gentle movements in chair yoga boost blood flow, which supports cardiovascular health and reduces swelling in extremities. It also helps lubricate joints, alleviating pain and stiffness caused by arthritis or inactivity.

6. Mental Clarity and Focus

Chair yoga incorporates mindfulness and meditation, which can enhance cognitive function, improve memory, and increase focus—key components of maintaining mental sharpness with age.

How Chair Yoga Supports Aging Gracefully

Aging gracefully doesn't just mean looking young; it's about feeling vibrant, staying active, and finding joy in everyday life. Chair yoga supports these goals in the following ways:

1. Accessibility and Adaptability

Unlike traditional yoga, chair yoga is accessible to individuals of all fitness levels and abilities. Whether dealing with chronic pain, reduced mobility, or fatigue, seniors can adapt poses to suit their unique needs.

2. Holistic Approach to Wellness

Chair yoga addresses physical, mental, and emotional health simultaneously. By combining movement, breath, and mindfulness, it helps seniors embrace a balanced lifestyle that promotes long-term well-being.

3. Encourages Social Connections

Chair yoga classes often create opportunities for seniors to connect with others. These shared experiences can reduce feelings of isolation, fostering a sense of community and belonging.

4. A Sustainable Fitness Option

Unlike high-impact exercises, chair yoga can be practiced daily without putting stress on the body. Its gentle nature ensures it's sustainable, making it an excellent lifelong fitness routine.

Getting Started: What You Need for a Successful Practice

Beginning your chair yoga journey is simple, but a few essentials can enhance your experience and ensure safety and comfort:

1. The Right Chair

Choose a sturdy, straight-backed chair without wheels or armrests. It should provide a stable base for seated poses and allow for comfortable movement. Place the chair on a non-slip surface to prevent sliding.

2. Comfortable Clothing

Wear loose, breathable clothing that allows for free movement. Avoid tight waistbands or restrictive fabrics that might hinder your stretches.

3. Supportive Props

For added support, consider using props like a small cushion for lumbar support or a rolled-up towel under the feet to ensure proper posture during poses.

4. A Quiet, Safe Space

Find a clutter-free space with enough room to stretch your arms and legs without restrictions. A calm environment will help you focus and enjoy the mindfulness aspects of chair yoga.

5. A Positive Mindset

Approach chair yoga with an open heart and patience. Each session is an opportunity to listen to your body, celebrate small victories, and progress at your own pace.

6. Optional: A Yoga Mat for Stability

Placing the chair on a yoga mat can provide extra stability, especially if you'll be incorporating standing poses using the chair for support.

By starting with these simple preparations, you'll set yourself up for a rewarding chair yoga experience that enhances your health, uplifts your spirit, and helps you age gracefully.

Chapter 1: Understanding Chair Yoga

Chair yoga is a gentle yet transformative practice that makes the benefits of yoga accessible to everyone, regardless of age, mobility, or fitness level. It adapts traditional yoga poses to be performed while seated or with the support of a chair, providing a safe and comfortable way to improve flexibility, strength, and mental well-being. In this chapter, we'll explore the essence of chair yoga, its key principles, how it differs from traditional yoga, and the central role of breath and mindfulness in the practice.

What is Chair Yoga?

Chair yoga is a modified form of yoga designed to meet the needs of individuals who may find traditional yoga poses challenging or inaccessible. By using a chair as a supportive prop, participants can perform a wide range of poses and stretches, whether seated or standing with the chair for balance.

Chair yoga focuses on:

- **Gentle Movements**: Slow and controlled motions to enhance mobility and reduce stiffness.

- **Accessibility**: Suitable for seniors, people with limited mobility, or those recovering from injuries.

- **Holistic Wellness**: A combination of physical activity, mindful breathing, and relaxation techniques.

This approach makes yoga not only feasible but also enjoyable for individuals who might otherwise feel excluded from traditional yoga practices.

The Key Principles Behind Chair Yoga

Chair yoga is grounded in the same principles as traditional yoga, adapted to meet the unique needs of its practitioners. Here are the core principles:

1. Inclusivity

Chair yoga embraces the idea that yoga is for everyone. It removes barriers, ensuring that individuals with physical limitations or chronic conditions can participate fully.

2. Mind-Body Connection

Like traditional yoga, chair yoga emphasizes the connection between the mind and body. Every movement is linked to the breath, creating a sense of harmony and balance.

3. Adaptability

Chair yoga is highly adaptable, with poses that can be modified to suit individual abilities. This flexibility ensures that each person can practice at their own pace and comfort level.

4. Safety and Comfort

Safety is a priority in chair yoga. By using a stable chair, participants can perform poses without the risk of falling or straining their bodies.

5. Progression

Chair yoga encourages gradual improvement. Over time, participants may notice increased strength, flexibility, and confidence, empowering them to explore more challenging variations.

Differences Between Traditional Yoga and Chair Yoga

While chair yoga retains the essence of traditional yoga, there are significant differences that make it more accessible and beginner-friendly:

Aspect	Traditional yoga	Chair yoga
Physical demands	Involves full-body poses and transitions like standing, balancing and floor work.	Focuses on seated or chair-supported poses, minimizing strain.

Accessibil ity	May require significant flexibility, strength or balance.	Designed for individuals with limited mobility or chronic conditions .
Props	May use props like blocks, straps, or bolsters.	The chair serves as the primary prop for support and stability.
Audience	Typically practiced by those with moderate to high levels of	Suitable for seniors, beginners, and individuals recovering

	fitness.	from injuries.

Chair yoga's unique approach allows participants to enjoy the mental and physical benefits of yoga without needing to perform challenging poses or transitions.

The Role of Breath and Mindfulness in Chair Yoga

Breathing and mindfulness are the foundation of any yoga practice, including chair yoga. These elements help deepen the mind-body connection and amplify the benefits of the physical movements.

1. The Power of Breath (Pranayama)

Breathing exercises in chair yoga play a vital role in:

- **Calming the Mind**: Deep breathing activates the parasympathetic nervous system, reducing stress and anxiety.

- **Improving Oxygen Flow:** Proper breathing enhances circulation and supports overall energy levels.

- **Supporting Movement**: Synchronizing breath with movement helps improve focus, coordination, and ease of motion.

Common breathing techniques in chair yoga include:

- **Abdominal Breathing**: Deep breaths into the diaphragm for relaxation.

- **Alternate Nostril Breathing**: Balancing energy and calming the mind.

- **Ocean Breath (Ujjayi)**: Creating a rhythmic and soothing breath pattern.

2. Mindfulness in Motion

Mindfulness is the practice of being fully present in the moment. In chair yoga, mindfulness enhances the practice by:

- Encouraging participants to focus on their breath and movements.

- Helping release mental clutter and promote clarity.

- Creating a sense of gratitude and awareness for one's body.

By integrating mindfulness, chair yoga becomes more than physical exercise—it becomes a meditative practice that nurtures mental and emotional health.

Chair yoga is a transformative practice that makes yoga accessible to individuals of all abilities. By understanding its principles, differences from traditional yoga, and the importance of breath and mindfulness, seniors can confidently embrace chair yoga as a way to enhance their physical, mental, and emotional well-being. This practice not only supports aging gracefully but also empowers individuals to stay active, engaged, and connected to their inner selves.

Chapter 2: Preparing for Your Practice

Preparation is the key to a safe, effective, and enjoyable chair yoga experience. Before you begin, it's essential to create an environment that promotes focus, comfort, and relaxation. This chapter will guide you through the essentials, from choosing the right chair to setting up a calming space, performing warm-up techniques, and embracing mindfulness as the foundation of your practice.

Choosing the Right Chair: What to Look For

The chair is the cornerstone of your chair yoga practice, acting as both a prop and a support system. Selecting the right chair ensures safety, stability, and ease of movement. Here's what to consider:

1. Stability and Sturdiness

- Choose a chair with a strong frame, ideally made of wood or metal, to prevent tipping or wobbling.

- Avoid chairs with wheels or swivel features, as they can reduce stability.

2. Seat Height and Depth

- The chair should allow your feet to rest flat on the ground, with your knees at a 90-degree angle.

- The seat should be deep enough to support your thighs but not so deep that it forces you to slouch.

3. Back Support

- A chair with a straight, firm back provides the best support for proper posture.

- Cushioned chairs are fine, but avoid overly soft or sinking seats.

4. Armrests (Optional)

- While armrests can offer additional support, they may limit your range of motion during certain poses. Consider a chair without armrests for maximum versatility.

By investing in the right chair, you'll create a secure foundation for your practice, allowing you to focus on movement and mindfulness without distractions.

Creating a Comfortable Space for Yoga

A well-prepared space can enhance your yoga experience by fostering calm and concentration. Here's how to set up your yoga sanctuary:

1. Find a Quiet, Clutter-Free Area

- Choose a space free from noise and distractions, such as a corner of a room or a shaded patio.

- Remove clutter to create an open, inviting environment.

2. Ensure Proper Lighting and Ventilation

- Natural light can create a serene atmosphere, but soft artificial lighting works well too.

- Good ventilation keeps the space fresh and energizing.

3. Use a Yoga Mat for Stability

- Placing your chair on a yoga mat prevents slipping, especially if your flooring is smooth or tiled.

4. Add Comfort Enhancements

- A small cushion or rolled towel can support your lower back or feet if needed.

- Keep a water bottle and a light blanket nearby for hydration and warmth during relaxation phases.

5. Personalize Your Space

- Add calming elements like candles, plants, or soothing

music to make the environment inviting and peaceful.

Creating a dedicated space sets the tone for a focused and rewarding chair yoga session.

Essential Warm-Up Techniques for Safe Movement

Warming up is vital to prepare your body for movement, reduce stiffness, and prevent injury. These gentle warm-ups are specifically tailored for chair yoga:

1. Neck Rolls

- Sit tall with your shoulders relaxed.

- Slowly lower your chin to your chest, then gently roll your head in a circular motion.

- Repeat in both directions to release tension in the neck and shoulders.

2. Shoulder Shrugs

- Lift your shoulders toward your ears as you inhale, then release them back down as you exhale.

- Repeat 5–10 times to loosen tight shoulder muscles.

3. Seated Cat-Cow Stretch

- Sit near the edge of your chair with your hands on your knees.

- On an inhale, arch your back and lift your chest (Cow Pose).

- On an exhale, round your back and tuck your chin to your chest (Cat Pose).

- Repeat for 5–8 breaths to stretch the spine and improve flexibility.

4. Ankle Rolls

- Lift one foot slightly off the floor and rotate your ankle in circular motions.

- Repeat in both directions, then switch to the other foot.

- This improves circulation and warms up the lower legs.

5. Gentle Seated Twists

- Place one hand on the opposite knee and the other on the chair's backrest.

- Inhale as you lengthen your spine, and exhale as you gently twist toward the backrest.

- Hold for a few breaths, then switch sides to warm up the spine and core.

A proper warm-up primes your body for movement and ensures a safe, enjoyable session.

How to Listen to Your Body and Practice Mindfulness

Chair yoga is not about pushing limits or achieving perfection; it's about tuning in to your body's needs and responding with care and awareness. Here's how to cultivate mindfulness during your practice:

1. Pay Attention to Sensations

- Notice how each movement feels—whether it's a stretch, a release, or a point of tension.

- If something feels uncomfortable or painful, ease out of the pose and modify as needed.

2. Stay Present

- Focus on your breath and the movements you're performing.

- If your mind starts to wander, gently bring your attention back to the present moment.

3. Practice Gratitude

- Acknowledge the effort your body is making and celebrate small victories.

- Gratitude fosters positivity and enhances the joy of practicing yoga.

4. Embrace Your Own Pace

- Yoga is a personal journey, and progress looks different for everyone.

- Avoid comparing yourself to others and focus on your own growth and comfort.

5. Use the Breath as an Anchor

- Breathe deeply and evenly throughout your practice.

- The breath helps you stay grounded, calm, and connected to your body.

Mindfulness transforms chair yoga into a meditative experience, allowing you to nurture both your body and mind.

Proper preparation is the foundation of a successful chair yoga practice. By selecting the right chair, creating a serene space, warming up effectively, and practicing mindfulness, you set the stage for a rewarding experience. These steps not only enhance safety and comfort but also help you cultivate a deeper connection with yourself, making every session a meaningful part of your journey to health and well-being.

Chapter 3: Chair Yoga Poses for Flexibility and Mobility

Flexibility and mobility are essential components of maintaining physical independence and ease of movement as we age. Chair yoga offers a gentle yet effective way to improve these aspects through targeted poses that loosen tight muscles, enhance joint range of motion, and promote overall body awareness. This chapter introduces five accessible chair yoga poses designed to increase flexibility, relieve tension, and improve posture.

Gentle Neck Stretches

The neck is one of the most common areas where tension builds, often leading to stiffness and discomfort. Gentle neck stretches help release tension and improve flexibility in the neck and shoulders.

How to Practice:

1. Sit tall in your chair with both feet flat on the ground and your hands resting on your thighs.

2. Slowly lower your right ear toward your right shoulder, keeping your shoulders relaxed.

3. Hold this position for 3–5 breaths, feeling the stretch along the left side of your neck.

4. Return to the center and repeat on the left side.

Variation:

- For a deeper stretch, place your right hand gently on the left side of your head and apply light pressure.

Benefits:

- Relieves tension in the neck and shoulders.

- Improves range of motion in the neck.

- Reduces stress and promotes relaxation.

Shoulder Openers for Tension Relief

Tight shoulders can restrict upper-body movement and cause discomfort. Shoulder openers improve flexibility and relieve tension in the shoulder area.

How to Practice:

1. Sit upright with your feet flat on the floor and your back away from the chair's backrest.

2. Inhale and lift your shoulders toward your ears.

3. Exhale and roll your shoulders back and down in a circular motion.

4. Repeat this motion 5–8 times.

Variation:

- Interlace your fingers behind your back, straighten your arms, and lift them slightly to open your chest and shoulders.

Benefits:

- Loosens tight shoulder muscles.

- Improves posture by opening the chest.

- Reduces stress and tension.

Spine Twists for Better Posture

Spinal twists enhance spinal flexibility, promote better posture, and stimulate digestion. They also relieve tension in the back and shoulders.

How to Practice:

1. Sit near the edge of your chair with both feet firmly on the ground.

2. Place your right hand on the outer edge of your left knee and your left hand on the chair's backrest.

3. Inhale and lengthen your spine.

4. Exhale and gently twist to the left, turning your gaze over your left shoulder.

5. Hold for 3-5 breaths, then return to the center.

6. Repeat on the other side.

Variation:

- For a gentler twist, keep your gaze forward instead of turning your head.

Benefits:

- Enhances spinal flexibility and mobility.

- Improves posture by aligning the spine.

- Stimulates internal organs, aiding digestion.

Side Stretches to Open the Hips and Chest

Side stretches target the obliques, open the chest, and improve flexibility in the hips and lower back. These stretches also promote better breathing by expanding the rib cage.

How to Practice:

1. Sit tall in your chair with your feet flat on the floor.

2. Place your left hand on the chair seat for support.

3. Inhale and lift your right arm overhead, reaching toward the ceiling.

4. Exhale and lean gently to the left, feeling the stretch along your right side.

5. Hold for 3–5 breaths, then return to the center.

6. Repeat on the other side.

Variation:

- Add a gentle twist by turning your gaze toward your raised hand.

Benefits:

- Stretches the sides of the torso and the hips.

- Opens the chest, promoting better posture and breathing.

- Relieves tension in the lower back.

Seated Forward Bends for Hamstring Flexibility

Hamstring flexibility is crucial for maintaining mobility and preventing lower back strain. Seated forward bends provide a gentle stretch for the hamstrings and the lower back.

How to Practice:

1. Sit near the edge of your chair with your feet hip-width apart and flat on the ground.

2. Straighten your legs slightly, keeping your heels on the floor and toes pointing up.

3. Inhale and lengthen your spine.

4. Exhale and hinge forward from your hips, reaching your hands toward your knees, shins, or toes (depending on your flexibility).

5. Keep your back straight and avoid rounding your shoulders.

6. Hold for 3–5 breaths, then slowly return to an upright position.

Variation:

- Use a yoga strap or towel looped around your feet for added support if reaching forward feels challenging.

Benefits:

- Stretches the hamstrings and calves.

- Relieves tension in the lower back.

- Promotes better flexibility and posture.

Chair yoga poses for flexibility and mobility are powerful tools for maintaining physical independence and comfort. Gentle neck stretches, shoulder openers, spine twists, side stretches, and seated forward bends work together to release tension, improve range of motion, and promote overall well-being. By practicing these poses regularly, you can enhance your flexibility and mobility while fostering a sense of calm and balance in your daily life.

Chapter 4: Strength and Balance Through Chair Yoga

As we age, maintaining strength and balance becomes crucial for preventing falls, staying mobile, and enhancing overall independence. Chair yoga provides a safe and accessible way to build strength in key muscle groups and improve balance, even for those with limited mobility. This chapter introduces a series of chair yoga poses designed to target lower body strength, core stability, and balance.

Seated Leg Lifts for Lower Body Strength

Strong leg muscles are essential for activities like walking, climbing stairs, and standing from a seated position. Seated leg lifts strengthen the quadriceps, hip flexors, and lower abdominal muscles.

How to Practice:

1. Sit tall in your chair with your feet flat on the ground and your hands resting on the sides of the chair.

2. Extend your right leg straight out, keeping your toes pointed upward.

3. Hold the leg in the air for 3–5 seconds, engaging your thigh and core muscles.

4. Slowly lower the leg back down without letting it touch the ground.

5. Repeat 8–10 times, then switch to the left leg.

Variation:

- For added intensity, attach ankle weights or hold the leg up for a longer duration.

Benefits:

- Strengthens the quadriceps and hip flexors.

- Improves lower body stability and mobility.

- Enhances core engagement.

Seated Warrior Poses to Improve Posture

The Warrior poses, adapted for a chair, are excellent for building strength in the arms, shoulders, and legs while promoting better posture and stability.

How to Practice Seated Warrior I:

1. Sit sideways on your chair, with your right hip against the backrest and your feet flat on the floor.

2. Extend your left leg back, keeping the sole of your foot flat on the floor or the toes pointed back.

3. Lift your arms overhead, palms facing each other, and gaze forward.

4. Hold for 3–5 breaths, feeling the stretch in your hips and the strength in your legs and arms.

5. Switch sides and repeat.

How to Practice Seated Warrior II:

1. Sit sideways on the chair as above, but this time, extend your arms out to the sides at shoulder height.

2. Keep your front knee bent at a 90-degree angle and your back leg extended straight.

3. Turn your gaze over your front hand.

4. Hold for 3–5 breaths, then switch sides.

Benefits:

- Strengthens the arms, shoulders, and legs.

- Opens the chest and promotes better posture.

- Enhances stability and balance.

Chair Poses to Strengthen Core Muscles

A strong core is the foundation for good balance, posture, and overall mobility. Chair yoga offers several poses to target core muscles safely and effectively.

How to Practice:

1. Sit upright with your back away from the chair's backrest and your feet flat on the floor.

2. Place your hands on your thighs for support.

3.   Engage   your   abdominal
muscles and lean back slightly,
keeping your spine straight.

4. Hold this position for 5–10
seconds,   then   return   to   an
upright position.

5. Repeat 8–10 times.

Variation:

- For added challenge, lift one or
  both feet off the ground while
  leaning back.

Benefits:

- Strengthens the abdominal and
  lower back muscles.

- Improves posture and spinal support.

- Enhances balance and stability.

Standing with Support: Building Balance and Stability

Practicing standing poses with the support of a chair improves balance, strengthens the lower body, and boosts confidence in everyday movements.

How to Practice:

1. Stand behind your chair, holding the backrest for support.

2. Shift your weight onto your left foot and slowly lift your right foot off the ground.

3. Hold the position for 5-10 seconds, focusing on engaging your core and maintaining balance.

4. Lower the right foot and switch to the left side.

Variation:

- For additional challenge, extend the lifted leg out to the side or back while keeping your balance.

Benefits:

- Enhances balance and stability.

- Strengthens the lower body and core.

- Builds confidence in standing and walking movements.

Chair Squats for Leg Strength

Chair squats are an effective way to build strength in the thighs, hips, and glutes while improving balance and coordination.

How to Practice:

1. Stand in front of your chair, with your feet shoulder-width apart and your knees slightly bent.

2. Lower yourself slowly as if you are going to sit in the chair, but stop just before your hips touch the seat.

3. Pause for a moment, then press through your heels to return to a standing position.

4. Repeat 8-10 times, keeping your movements slow and controlled.

Variation:

- Use the chair's armrests for added support if needed.

Benefits:

- Strengthens the thighs, hips, and glutes.

- Improves balance and coordination.

- Enhances mobility for everyday activities like sitting and standing.

Chair yoga offers a safe and effective way to build strength and balance, key components of healthy aging. From seated leg lifts to chair squats, these poses target specific muscle groups while improving overall stability and confidence. By incorporating these exercises into your routine, you'll support your physical independence, reduce the risk of falls, and enjoy a greater sense of control over your body. Embrace the journey toward strength and balance with chair yoga as your guide.

Chapter 5: Relaxation and Stress Relief

In our fast-paced world, stress and tension can accumulate in both the mind and body, leading to a range of physical and emotional challenges. Relaxation and stress relief are vital components of a balanced lifestyle, especially for seniors, as they promote better sleep, lower blood pressure, and overall well-being. Chair yoga offers accessible and effective ways to calm the mind, release tension, and restore a sense of peace. In this chapter, we'll explore techniques and poses to help you unwind, reduce stress, and nurture relaxation.

Gentle Breathing Techniques for Relaxation

Controlled breathing is a cornerstone of yoga and relaxation practices. Gentle breathing techniques can help calm the nervous system, lower stress hormones, and enhance mindfulness.

How to Practice: Belly Breathing (Diaphragmatic Breathing):

1. Sit comfortably in your chair with your feet flat on the ground.

2. Place one hand on your chest and the other on your belly.

3. Inhale deeply through your nose, allowing your belly to rise while keeping your chest still.

4. Exhale slowly through your mouth, feeling your belly contract gently.

5. Repeat for 5–10 breaths, focusing on the rhythm of your breath.

Variation:

- Add a count to your breath (e.g., inhale for 4 counts, exhale for 6 counts) to deepen relaxation.

Benefits:

- Reduces stress and anxiety.

- Enhances focus and mindfulness.

- Promotes better oxygen exchange and lung capacity.

Guided Meditation for Stress Reduction

Meditation is a powerful tool for calming the mind, fostering self-awareness, and reducing stress. Guided meditations provide a structured way to focus and relax.

How to Practice:

1. Sit comfortably with your hands resting on your thighs and close your eyes.

2. Focus on your breath, noticing the natural rhythm of inhalation and exhalation.

3. In your mind, visualize a peaceful scene, such as a beach, forest, or garden.

4. Imagine the sounds, scents, and sensations of this serene place.

5. Stay in this visualization for 5-10 minutes, returning your focus to your breath whenever your mind wanders.

Variation:

- Use a recorded guided meditation or soothing music to enhance your experience.

Benefits:

- Reduces stress and improves mental clarity.

- Promotes a sense of calm and inner peace.

- Supports emotional resilience.

Seated Child's Pose for Deep Rest

The Child's Pose is a restorative yoga posture that helps relax the back, shoulders, and neck while calming the mind. Adapting it for a chair makes it accessible for seniors.

How to Practice:

1. Sit near the edge of your chair with your feet flat on the floor, hip-width apart.

2. Inhale and lengthen your spine.

3. Exhale and slowly hinge forward from your hips, letting your torso rest on your thighs.

4. Allow your arms to hang down toward the floor or rest them on your knees.

5. Stay in this position for 5–10 breaths, breathing deeply and relaxing into the stretch.

Variation:

- Place a pillow on your thighs to support your upper body for added comfort.

Benefits:

- Relieves tension in the lower back and shoulders.

- Encourages deep relaxation and rest.

- Calms the nervous system and reduces stress.

Progressive Muscle Relaxation While Seated

Progressive muscle relaxation (PMR) involves tensing and releasing muscle groups to reduce physical tension and foster relaxation. This technique is highly effective for managing stress.

How to Practice:

1. Sit comfortably in your chair with your feet flat on the floor.

2. Begin with your feet: Inhale and tense the muscles in your feet for 5 seconds.

3. Exhale and release the tension completely.

4. Move upward through your body, tensing and relaxing your calves, thighs, abdomen, arms, shoulders, and neck.

5. End with your face, tensing and releasing your jaw, cheeks, and forehead.

Variation:

- Combine PMR with gentle breathing for an even deeper sense of relaxation.

Benefits:

- Relieves physical tension and stress.

- Increases body awareness.

- Promotes a state of calm and tranquility.

The Power of Gratitude and Positive Thinking

Cultivating gratitude and a positive mindset can profoundly impact emotional well-being and resilience. By focusing on the positive aspects of life, we can shift our perspective and reduce stress.

How to Practice:

1. Sit quietly and reflect on three things you are grateful for. These could be as simple as a sunny

day, a kind word from a friend, or your ability to practice yoga.

2. Write these down in a gratitude journal or say them aloud.

3. Practice affirmations by repeating positive phrases such as, "I am calm, I am strong, I am at peace."

Variation:

- Pair gratitude practice with your breathing exercises for a more holistic approach.

Benefits:

- Reduces stress and anxiety.

- Fosters a positive outlook on life.

- Enhances emotional resilience and well-being.

Relaxation and stress relief are essential components of a healthy and balanced life, particularly as we age. Through gentle breathing, guided meditation, restorative poses like Seated Child's Pose, and techniques like progressive muscle relaxation, chair yoga provides practical tools to calm the mind and ease physical tension. Embracing gratitude and positive thinking further enriches this practice, creating a more peaceful and joyful state of being. By incorporating these relaxation techniques into your daily routine, you can cultivate a sense of calm and resilience, no matter what challenges life may bring.

Chapter 6: Chair Yoga for Common Ailments

Chair yoga is a gentle yet effective way to address many common ailments experienced by seniors, such as back pain, arthritis, poor digestion, joint stiffness, and circulation issues. By tailoring movements to specific needs, chair yoga provides a safe and accessible approach to finding relief and improving overall well-being. This chapter will guide you through targeted poses and techniques designed to alleviate discomfort and promote better health.

Relieving Back Pain with Simple Movements

Back pain is a common concern among seniors, often caused by poor posture, muscle imbalances, or sedentary lifestyles. Chair yoga can help stretch and strengthen the back, relieving pain and improving posture.

Seated Cat-Cow Stretch:

1. Sit tall with your feet flat on the floor and hands on your knees.

2. Inhale as you arch your back, lifting your chest and tilting your pelvis forward (Cow Pose).

3. Exhale as you round your spine, tucking your chin to your chest and drawing your belly button inward (Cat Pose).

4. Repeat this flow for 5–10 breaths, moving gently and rhythmically.

Benefits:

- Eases tension in the spine and back muscles.

- Improves flexibility and posture.

- Stimulates spinal mobility and alignment.

Managing Arthritis with Chair Yoga

Arthritis can cause joint pain, stiffness, and inflammation, limiting mobility. Chair yoga offers gentle movements to improve joint flexibility, reduce stiffness, and increase circulation to affected areas.

Seated Finger and Wrist Stretches:

1. Extend your arms in front of you at shoulder height.

2. Slowly open and close your fingers, spreading them wide as you open and curling them tightly into a fist as you close.

3. Circle your wrists clockwise and counterclockwise for 5–10 repetitions each.

Seated Knee Lifts:

1. Sit with your back straight and hands resting on the chair for support.

2. Inhale and lift your right knee toward your chest as high as comfortable.

3. Exhale and lower it back to the ground.

4. Repeat 5–10 times per leg.

- Reduces stiffness in fingers, wrists, knees, and other joints.

- Improves range of motion and flexibility.

- Promotes joint lubrication and circulation.

Yoga for Improved Digestion

Digestive issues like bloating, constipation, and indigestion can be improved with gentle yoga poses that stimulate the abdominal organs and encourage movement within the digestive system.

Seated Twist:

1. Sit tall with your feet flat on the floor.

2. Place your right hand on the back of your chair and your left hand on your right thigh.

3. Inhale to lengthen your spine, and exhale as you twist gently to the right.

4. Hold for 3-5 breaths, then return to center and repeat on the left side.

Seated Forward Fold:

1. Sit with your feet hip-width apart.

2. Inhale and lengthen your spine.

3. Exhale as you hinge forward from your hips, letting your torso rest on your thighs and your hands dangle toward the floor.

4. Breathe deeply for 3–5 breaths, then slowly rise back up.

Benefits:

- Stimulates digestion and alleviates bloating.

- Massages internal organs for improved gut function.

- Relieves tension in the abdomen.

Easing Joint Stiffness and Muscle Tension

Joint stiffness and muscle tension can limit mobility and cause discomfort. Chair yoga helps release tightness and improve flexibility through gentle stretches and movements.

Seated Shoulder Rolls:

- 1. Sit tall with your hands resting on your thighs.

  2. Inhale as you roll your shoulders up toward your ears.

3. Exhale as you roll them back and down.

4. Repeat 8–10 times, then reverse the direction.

Seated Hamstring Stretch:

- 1. Sit on the edge of your chair with one leg extended straight out, heel resting on the floor.

- 2. Inhale to lengthen your spine, and exhale as you hinge forward slightly, feeling a stretch along the back of your extended leg.

- 3. Hold for 3–5 breaths, then switch legs.

Benefits:

- Relieves tension in the shoulders, back, and legs.

- Improves flexibility in tight muscles.

- Increases joint mobility and reduces stiffness.

Techniques for Enhancing Circulation

Good circulation is essential for overall health, as it delivers oxygen and nutrients to tissues and helps remove waste products. Chair yoga encourages better blood flow, particularly in the extremities.

Ankle Rolls and Toe Taps:

- 1. Sit with your feet flat on the floor.

  2. Lift one foot slightly off the ground and circle your ankle clockwise and counterclockwise for 5–10 repetitions.

  3. Lower your foot and tap your toes on the floor several times.

  4. Repeat with the other foot.

Seated Leg Pumps:

- 1. Sit tall with your feet flat on the ground.

2. Inhale and lift your heels off the floor, coming onto your toes.

3. Exhale and lower your heels back down.

4. Repeat this movement for 10–15 repetitions.

Benefits:

- Improves circulation to the legs, feet, and hands.

- Reduces swelling and prevents blood pooling in the lower extremities.

- Enhances energy and reduces fatigue.

Chair yoga provides targeted and effective solutions for managing common ailments such as back pain, arthritis, poor digestion, joint stiffness, and circulation problems. By incorporating these gentle movements into your daily routine, you can alleviate discomfort, enhance mobility, and promote better overall health. With consistent practice, chair yoga becomes a powerful tool for aging gracefully and living life with greater ease and comfort.

Chapter 7: Chair Yoga for Mental Clarity and Focus

As we age, maintaining mental clarity and focus becomes increasingly important. Chair yoga offers a holistic approach to nurturing mental health, combining breathwork, gentle movement, and mindfulness to improve memory, reduce stress, and enhance emotional well-being. In this chapter, you'll discover how chair yoga can support mental clarity, emotional balance, and resilience.

Breathing Techniques to Clear the Mind

Breathing is the foundation of yoga and plays a critical role in calming the mind, reducing distractions, and improving focus. Chair yoga includes accessible breathing techniques that seniors can easily incorporate into their daily lives.

1. **Alternate Nostril Breathing (Nadi Shodhana):**

> 1. Sit tall with your feet flat on the floor.
>
> 2. Use your right thumb to gently close your right nostril.
>
> 3. Inhale deeply through your left nostril.
>
> 4. Close your left nostril with your ring finger, release your right nostril, and exhale fully through the right nostril.

5.   Repeat   the   process, alternating sides, for 5–10 cycles.

2.   Three-Part   Breath   (Dirga Pranayama):

1. Sit comfortably with your hands resting on your thighs.

2. Inhale deeply, first filling your lower belly, then your ribcage, and finally your upper chest.

3. Exhale slowly in reverse order, releasing from your chest, ribcage, and belly.

4. Repeat for 5–10 breaths, focusing on the flow of air.

- Clears mental fog and sharpens focus.

- Balances energy levels and promotes relaxation.

- Enhances oxygen supply to the brain for improved cognitive function.

Yoga for Memory and Cognitive Function

Chair yoga enhances memory and cognitive function by improving blood flow to the brain and reducing stress, which can impair mental performance. Simple movements combined with mindfulness can help seniors stay mentally sharp.

1. Seated Cross-Crawl:

1. Sit tall with your feet flat on the floor.

2. Lift your right knee while tapping it with your left hand.

3. Lower your leg and repeat on the opposite side, lifting your left knee and tapping it with your right hand.

4. Continue alternating for 10–15 repetitions.

2. Brain-Boosting Twist:

1. Sit with your feet flat on the ground and your hands on your thighs.

2. Inhale to lengthen your spine, and exhale as you twist gently to the right, looking over your shoulder.

3. Inhale to return to center, and exhale to twist to the left.

4. Repeat for 5–8 cycles, focusing on the movement and your breath.

Benefits:

- Enhances coordination and brain-body connection.

- Stimulates neural pathways to support memory retention.

- Promotes mental alertness and reduces sluggishness.

Meditation Practices for Mental Wellness

Meditation is a key component of yoga that fosters mental peace and emotional resilience. Chair yoga includes simple, seated meditation techniques that encourage mindfulness and reduce stress.

1. Guided Visualization:

1. Sit comfortably with your hands resting on your lap.

2. Close your eyes and take a few deep breaths.

3. Visualize a calming place, such as a peaceful beach or a serene garden.

4. Imagine yourself immersed in this place, noticing the sounds, smells, and sensations.

5. Stay in this visualization for 5–10 minutes, then slowly open your eyes.

2. Mantra Meditation:

1. Choose a calming word or phrase, such as "peace" or "I am calm."

2. Sit comfortably with your spine straight and your hands resting on your lap.

3. Close your eyes and silently repeat the mantra with each breath.

4. Continue for 5–10 minutes, focusing on the rhythm of the mantra.

Benefits:

- Reduces stress and promotes relaxation.

- Improves concentration and emotional balance.

- Encourages a deeper connection to the present moment.

Boosting Mood and Reducing Anxiety with Yoga

Chair yoga provides natural techniques for reducing anxiety and boosting mood by combining physical movement with mindful breathing. These practices stimulate the release of endorphins and reduce cortisol levels, promoting a sense of calm and happiness.

1. Seated Sun Salutations:

1. Inhale as you sweep your arms overhead.

2. Exhale as you fold forward, bringing your hands toward your feet.

3. Inhale as you rise back to a seated position with your arms overhead.

4. Exhale as you lower your hands to your lap.

5. Repeat 5–8 times, moving gently with your breath.

2. Heart-Opening Pose:

1. Sit tall with your hands clasped behind your back.

2. Inhale as you gently lift your chest and open your shoulders.

3. Exhale as you release the stretch.

4. Repeat 5–8 times, focusing on creating a sense of openness and positivity.

Benefits:

- Alleviates symptoms of anxiety and depression.

- Promotes emotional well-being and relaxation.

- Enhances self-awareness and self-compassion.

Building Mental Resilience Through Regular Practice

Mental resilience is the ability to adapt to challenges and recover from stress. Regular chair yoga practice strengthens mental resilience by fostering a calm and centered mindset.

1. Grounding Practice:

1. Sit with your feet flat on the floor and your hands resting on your knees.

2. Close your eyes and take slow, deep breaths.

3. Visualize your feet rooted firmly into the ground, like the roots of a tree.

4. Stay with this visualization for 3–5 minutes, focusing on stability and strength.

2. Affirmation Practice:

1. Sit comfortably with your spine straight.

2. Close your eyes and repeat a positive affirmation, such as "I am strong and capable" or "I approach challenges with grace."

3. Repeat the affirmation silently or aloud for 3–5 minutes, allowing the words to resonate deeply.

- Builds emotional strength and adaptability.

- Encourages positive thinking and confidence.

- Helps seniors face challenges with a calm and focused mindset.

Chair yoga is a powerful tool for nurturing mental clarity, focus, and emotional resilience. By incorporating breathing techniques, gentle movements, and mindfulness practices, seniors can enhance their cognitive function, reduce stress, and cultivate a greater sense of well-being. Regular practice not only supports mental wellness but also fosters a positive and resilient approach to life's challenges. With chair yoga, you can embrace each day with a clear mind and a calm heart.

Chapter 8: Building a Daily Chair Yoga Routine

A daily chair yoga routine can transform your physical and mental well-being by fostering strength, flexibility, and relaxation in a way that is accessible and sustainable. This chapter provides a roadmap to design a personalized chair yoga routine, integrate it into your daily life, and maintain motivation for long-term benefits.

Designing a Personalized Routine for Your Needs

Creating a chair yoga routine tailored to your unique needs ensures you reap the most benefits while accommodating your physical abilities and goals.

1. Assess Your Goals:

- **Flexibility**: Focus on stretches that target tight muscles and joints.

- **Strength**: Incorporate poses that engage your core, legs, and arms.

- **Relaxation**: Include breathing exercises and meditative practices to reduce stress.

- **Balance**: Add exercises that improve stability and coordination.

2.   Consider   Your   Physical Limitations:

- Choose movements that feel comfortable and avoid anything that causes pain.

- Modify poses as needed with props such as cushions or straps.

- Consult a healthcare professional if you have any medical conditions.

3. Create a Balanced Sequence:

A well-rounded routine includes:

- **Warm-Up**: Gentle movements to prepare your body.

- **Strength Poses**: Build muscle and improve posture.

- **Flexibility Exercises**: Stretch and release tension.

- **Relaxation**: End with deep breathing or meditation.

Sample Routine:

1. **Warm-Up**: Neck rolls, shoulder shrugs, and seated side stretches (5 minutes).

2. **Strength**: Seated leg lifts, chair squats, and seated warrior poses (10 minutes).

3. Flexibility: Seated forward bends and gentle spine twists (10 minutes).

- **4. Relaxation**: Guided breathing or visualization (5 minutes).

How to Combine Strength, Flexibility, and Relaxation

A daily chair yoga routine should strike a balance between building strength, improving flexibility, and promoting relaxation.

1. Integrating Strength:

- Focus on exercises like seated leg lifts and chair poses to engage key muscle groups.

- Use your body weight to build endurance, targeting core stability and lower body strength.

2. Enhancing Flexibility:

- Incorporate dynamic stretches such as side stretches and spine twists to improve mobility.

- Practice slow, deep stretches that target areas prone to stiffness, like the hips, shoulders, and hamstrings.

3. Embracing Relaxation:

- Dedicate time to calming breathing techniques, such as alternate nostril breathing or three-part breath.

- Include a short meditation to center your mind and reduce stress.

- **Pro Tip**: Use music or nature sounds to create a calming environment and enhance your practice.

Tips for Staying Consistent and Motivated

Sticking to a daily chair yoga routine requires commitment and a few strategies to keep you motivated.

1. Set Realistic Goals:

- Start with 10–15 minutes a day and gradually increase the duration as you grow more comfortable.

- Set specific goals, like improving flexibility in your hamstrings or enhancing balance.

2. Make It Enjoyable:

- Choose a time of day when you feel most energized or relaxed.

- Wear comfortable clothing and use a supportive chair to enhance your experience.

3. Track Your Progress:

- Keep a journal to document your practice and note any improvements in strength, flexibility, or mood.

- Celebrate small victories, like mastering a pose or completing a week of consistent practice.

4. Find Support:

- Join a local chair yoga class or online community for encouragement and accountability.

- Share your journey with friends or family to inspire them to join.

5. Overcome Challenges:

- If you miss a day, don't be discouraged. Resume your routine the next day.

- On busy days, do a shorter practice or focus on one area, like breathing or stretching.

Integrating Chair Yoga into Your Day-to-Day Life

One of the greatest advantages of chair yoga is its accessibility and versatility. You can incorporate it seamlessly into your daily schedule.

1. Morning Routine:

- Begin your day with a 5-minute session of gentle stretches and deep breathing to wake up your body and mind.

2. Midday Break:

- Use chair yoga to release tension and boost energy during a lunch break or after prolonged sitting.

3. Evening Relaxation:

- Wind down with calming poses and meditation to prepare your body for restful sleep.

4. On the Go:

- Practice simple poses like seated side stretches or shoulder rolls while waiting in line or during travel.

5. Pair Yoga with Daily Tasks:

- Combine yoga with activities like reading or watching TV. For example, practice seated forward bends or leg lifts during commercials.

Building a daily chair yoga routine is a powerful way to nurture your physical and mental health while accommodating the unique needs of aging. By designing a personalized sequence, balancing strength, flexibility, and relaxation, and staying consistent, you can create a sustainable habit that enriches your life. With chair yoga, every day becomes an opportunity to move with purpose, stay mindful, and embrace a healthier, more vibrant version of yourself.

Chapter 9: Adapting Chair Yoga for Special Needs

Chair yoga offers a versatile and inclusive approach to wellness, making it accessible for individuals with a range of physical and health challenges. This chapter delves into the ways chair yoga can be adapted to suit specific needs, including limited mobility, chronic illnesses, recovery after surgery, and fatigue, while also exploring how caregivers can participate in the practice.

Chair Yoga for Those with Limited Mobility

Chair yoga provides an excellent way for individuals with limited mobility to experience the benefits of yoga without the need to move to the floor.

1. Focus on Accessible Movements:

- Prioritize small, gentle movements like wrist circles, ankle rolls, and shoulder shrugs.

- Encourage movements that enhance circulation and reduce stiffness, such as seated leg lifts or side stretches.

2. Support Through Props:

- Use additional support, such as pillows or towels, to enhance comfort and stability.

- Opt for chairs with armrests and a sturdy back for added balance.

3. Celebrate Progress:

- Small improvements in flexibility or strength are meaningful milestones.

- Encourage participants to focus on what they can do rather than what feels difficult.

Sample Poses:

- **Seated Cat-Cow Pose:** Gently mobilizes the spine and stretches the back.

- **Seated Forward Fold:** Encourages a gentle stretch in the hamstrings and back.

Modifications for People with Chronic Illnesses

Individuals with chronic conditions, such as arthritis, diabetes, or heart disease, can benefit greatly from chair yoga. Modifications ensure their practice is safe and effective.

1. Arthritis-Friendly Movements:

- Focus on low-impact poses to reduce joint pain and stiffness, such as seated twists and gentle hand stretches.

- Avoid poses that place excessive strain on inflamed joints.

2. Yoga for Heart Health:

- Incorporate slow, mindful breathing exercises to reduce stress and improve cardiovascular function.

- Avoid rapid movements or holding poses for extended periods.

3. Energy Management for Chronic Fatigue Syndrome:

- Opt for restorative poses and relaxation techniques to conserve energy.

- Keep sessions short, focusing on quality over quantity.

How to Safely Practice Chair Yoga After Surgery

Chair yoga can play a supportive role in post-surgery recovery, helping to rebuild strength and flexibility while promoting relaxation.

1. Consult Your Healthcare Provider:

- Always seek medical clearance before starting yoga after surgery.

- Discuss which movements are safe based on the type of surgery.

2. Emphasize Gentle Movements:

- Begin with subtle exercises like wrist and ankle rolls or deep breathing.

- Gradually progress to seated stretches and poses as your body heals.

3. Avoid Straining Surgical Areas:

- Be mindful of movements that could impact the surgical site or stitches.

- Use props to support gentle engagement of muscles without overexertion.

4. Focus on Relaxation:

- Include guided meditation or deep breathing to aid in stress reduction and recovery.

Encouraging Restorative Practices for Those with Fatigue

Fatigue, whether from chronic illness or stress, requires a gentle approach that prioritizes restoration over exertion. Chair yoga offers a way to recharge without overwhelming the body.

1. Restorative Poses:

- Include poses like the seated child's pose or seated forward bend for deep relaxation.

- Use props to support the body fully and reduce effort.

2. Gentle Breathing Techniques:

- Practice diaphragmatic breathing or alternate nostril breathing to promote relaxation.

- Keep breathing exercises short and soothing to prevent exhaustion.

3. Short and Simple Sessions:

- Limit sessions to 5–10 minutes if energy levels are low.

- Encourage participants to rest as needed during the practice.

Working with Caregivers: Yoga for Two

Chair yoga can be a shared experience between caregivers and those they support, fostering connection and mutual relaxation.

1. Partner Stretches:

- Try seated partner stretches, such as back-to-back breathing or side stretches, for shared movement.

- Encourage gentle stretches where one person provides light support, such as a seated forward fold with assistance.

2. Breathing Together:

- Practice synchronized breathing exercises to promote relaxation and bonding.

- Use simple breathing patterns, like inhaling for four counts and exhaling for four counts, to align breath rhythms.

3. Encourage Shared Mindfulness:

- Include guided meditations or gratitude exercises that both participants can enjoy.

- Focus on fostering a positive and calming environment.

4. Building Emotional Support:

- Caregivers can benefit from chair yoga by reducing their own stress levels.

- Encourage caregivers to participate fully, reminding them that self-care enhances their ability to care for others.

Adapting chair yoga for special needs ensures that individuals of all abilities and health conditions can experience the physical and mental benefits of yoga. By tailoring poses and techniques to specific circumstances, chair yoga becomes a powerful tool for improving quality of life, reducing discomfort, and fostering a sense of empowerment. Whether you're supporting recovery, managing a chronic condition, or practicing with a caregiver, chair yoga offers a pathway to wellness that is inclusive, restorative, and deeply enriching.

Chapter 10: Inspirational Stories from Seniors Who Practice Chair Yoga

Chair yoga isn't just about physical postures—it's about transformation. This chapter shares the inspiring stories of seniors who have integrated chair yoga into their lives, highlighting the real-life benefits they've experienced, the struggles they've overcome, and the wisdom they've gained. These stories prove that age is no barrier to starting a new journey toward improved health, greater mental clarity, and enhanced well-being.

Transformative Stories from Chair Yoga Practitioners

1. Jane's Journey: Overcoming Chronic Pain

Jane, a 72-year-old retired teacher, had been struggling with chronic back pain for years. Sitting for long periods or bending over to pick up objects became a daily challenge. After a doctor recommended chair yoga, Jane was hesitant, thinking it might not make a real difference. But after just a few weeks of practicing gentle movements and stretches, she noticed a significant reduction in her pain levels. Jane's transformation wasn't just physical; her sense of hope and well-being soared.

"Chair yoga has given me a new lease on life. I can move more freely, and I feel like I'm in control of my body again," says Jane. "The practice helps me listen to my body and work with it, not against it."

2. Bob's Story: Finding Balance After a Stroke

Bob, a 68-year-old man who had suffered a stroke a year prior, found his balance and coordination severely affected. Simple tasks like standing up or walking became overwhelming. His physical therapist suggested chair yoga as a way to regain strength and mobility while sitting. Bob began his journey with small movements—ankle circles and gentle stretches—before progressing to seated warrior poses and standing with support.

Now, nearly a year later, Bob's posture has improved, and he's regained strength in his legs and core. His balance has significantly improved, and he enjoys the freedom of walking without assistance.

"Chair yoga gave me back my independence. It's more than just physical exercise; it's a way to heal my mind too," Bob reflects. "The mental clarity I get from the practice is just as important as the physical benefits."

3. Maria's Path to Stress Relief and Relaxation

Maria, a 75-year-old grandmother, had been experiencing high levels of stress, worsened by caregiving for her elderly husband. Her energy levels were low, and sleep was often elusive.

One day, a fellow caregiver recommended chair yoga to help with relaxation. Maria was skeptical at first but decided to give it a try.

Through consistent practice, Maria discovered the power of deep breathing and meditation to release tension. The calming effect of chair yoga helped her sleep better and gave her the tools to manage stress. Now, Maria practices daily, finding peace and rejuvenation in her seated practice.

"Chair yoga has transformed my stress levels. I've learned to breathe through difficult moments and truly relax. It's a gift I give myself every day," says Maria.

Real-Life Benefits of a Regular Chair Yoga Practice

1. Physical Health Improvements

Seniors who practice chair yoga regularly report noticeable improvements in their physical health. From increased flexibility and mobility to improved posture and balance, chair yoga helps maintain functional independence. For many, it's the perfect way to stay active without the strain of traditional exercise.

- **Improved Circulation:** Chair yoga helps stimulate blood flow, reducing swelling and discomfort in the legs and feet.

- **Joint Pain Relief:** Gentle stretching and movements help keep joints limber, reducing stiffness and pain from arthritis or other joint conditions.

- **Strength Building**: Regular practice strengthens core muscles, arms, and legs, enhancing overall functional strength.

2. Mental and Emotional Well-Being

Chair yoga is as much about mental clarity as it is about physical movement. Seniors practicing chair yoga often report better mental health, including reduced anxiety and improved mood. This is due to the mindfulness, deep breathing, and relaxation techniques incorporated into every session.

- **Stress Reduction**: Breathing techniques and mindful movement help decrease the body's stress response, leading to a calmer, more centered state.

- **Increased Mental Clarity**: Practitioners experience improved focus, memory, and cognitive function as a result of the mental engagement required during yoga.

- **Emotional Balance**: The gentle practice of chair yoga fosters a sense of inner peace and self-compassion, contributing to emotional well-being.

3. Social and Community Benefits

Beyond physical and mental health improvements, chair yoga has provided many seniors with a sense of community. Whether practiced in group settings or online, chair yoga classes offer a space to meet others, share experiences, and feel supported. Many seniors report that the social connection provided through yoga enhances their overall quality of life.

Words of Wisdom from Experienced Chair Yoga Students

1. Advice from Betty: A Senior Advocate of Consistency

Betty, a 69-year-old yoga enthusiast, has been practicing chair yoga for over five years. Her biggest piece of advice for new students is consistency.

"It doesn't matter how long you practice, just practice every day. Even a few minutes of movement can make a big difference," Betty says. "It's not about being perfect; it's about showing up for yourself."

Betty believes in the power of small, consistent efforts to improve health over time, emphasizing that the benefits of chair yoga accumulate gradually.

2. Marcus' Wisdom: Embracing the Journey, Not the Destination

Marcus, 80, reflects on his experience with chair yoga as a reminder to be patient with oneself. Having been through a major surgery, he initially struggled with the idea of trying something new. He now feels stronger, more flexible, and more in tune with his body.

"Chair yoga has taught me that it's not about what I can or can't do— it's about showing up and embracing the journey," Marcus shares. "The most important thing is to listen to your body and work with it."

3. Linda's Words on Self-Care

Linda, 74, who began chair yoga after experiencing a major life change, shares how the practice has helped her focus on self-care.

"I spent so many years taking care of others, but chair yoga has shown me the importance of caring for myself. It's my time to relax, stretch, and just breathe. I feel so much better mentally and physically," says Linda.

Her advice to new practitioners? "Make yoga a part of your self-care routine, and don't be afraid to take it slow. You're worth it!"

The transformative stories shared in this chapter highlight the profound impact chair yoga can have on seniors. From physical health improvements and pain relief to emotional balance and a sense of community, the benefits of a regular chair yoga practice are wide-ranging. Seniors from all walks of life are discovering the power of mindful movement, breathing, and relaxation, proving that it's never too late to start a practice that nourishes the body, mind, and spirit. Through these inspirational stories, it's clear that chair yoga is not just a practice—it's a path to a healthier, more fulfilling life at any age.

Conclusion: Embracing the Journey and Moving Forward with Chair Yoga

As we reach the conclusion of this guide, it's important to reflect on the incredible potential that chair yoga holds for seniors. From the first step of learning the movements to the ultimate benefits of a consistent practice, chair yoga offers a holistic approach to well-being, enriching both body and mind. This is not just an exercise routine—it's a transformative journey that nurtures flexibility, strength, mental clarity, and emotional balance.

Embracing the Journey: The Lasting Benefits of Chair Yoga

Chair yoga is a lifelong practice that goes far beyond simply completing a set of movements. It is about embracing the journey of self-care, tuning into your body's signals, and fostering a deeper connection to your own health. Through the consistent practice of gentle movements, breathing techniques, and mindful postures, the lasting benefits of chair yoga unfold over time.

- **Improved Physical Health**: Whether you're focusing on strength, flexibility, or mobility, chair yoga allows you to target multiple aspects of your physical health. The gentle stretches and poses improve circulation, ease joint pain, and help alleviate common age-related ailments such as back pain and arthritis. By incorporating chair yoga into your routine, you're not only improving your body's functionality but also reducing the risk of injuries and maintaining your independence as you age.

Mental Clarity and Emotional Wellness: Chair yoga is an effective tool for reducing stress, enhancing cognitive function, and boosting mood. As you practice mindfulness and focus on your breath, you'll find that anxiety and mental fatigue diminish. The mental clarity that comes from a regular chair yoga practice promotes a sense of peace, while also offering tools to manage stress, depression, and anxiety.

- **Better Quality of Life**: Seniors who practice chair yoga report an overall improvement in their quality of life. From the relief of chronic pain to the ability to perform everyday tasks with greater ease, chair yoga supports a greater sense of well-being. It creates space for self-care and encourages a mindset of resilience and positivity, which is crucial for healthy aging.

Embracing chair yoga means embarking on a journey of self-discovery and improvement. Each practice is a step forward, bringing you closer to a balanced, fulfilled life.

Moving Forward: Keeping Yoga Part of Your Wellness Plan

Now that you've experienced the foundational elements of chair yoga, the next step is to continue integrating it into your daily wellness plan. To truly reap the full benefits, chair yoga should become an ongoing practice—a vital part of your routine. Here's how you can move forward:

1. **Set Realistic Goals**: Start by setting achievable goals that fit your lifestyle. Whether it's practicing for 10 minutes every morning, doing a chair yoga session before bed, or attending a class once a week, find a routine that works for you. Progress at your own pace, and

don't be afraid to adjust your goals as needed.

2. **Incorporate It Into Your Daily Life**: You don't have to reserve chair yoga just for your mat. Integrate small movements throughout the day—whether it's a seated stretch while watching TV or taking a few deep breaths while waiting for your coffee to brew. These little moments can help reinforce the benefits of yoga in your daily life.

3. **Join a Community**: Yoga is not only about the physical postures; it's also about connection. Joining a group or class—whether in person or

online—can offer support, motivation, and a sense of camaraderie. Practicing with others can enhance your sense of belonging, which plays a significant role in overall health and well-being.

4. **Listen to Your Body**: As you continue your journey with chair yoga, always listen to what your body is telling you. Don't push yourself too hard, and be mindful of any discomfort or pain. Over time, your body will become stronger and more flexible, but respect your limits, and modify poses as needed.

5. **Maintain Consistency**: The key to achieving lasting benefits from chair yoga is consistency. Regular practice, even if it's just a few minutes each day, will yield the greatest results. Make it a part of your routine and commit to honoring your practice as part of your wellness plan.

Moving forward with chair yoga means making it an integral part of your life. As you continue practicing, you'll experience a more profound sense of connection between your mind, body, and spirit, enhancing every aspect of your health.

Final Tips for a Lifelong Practice

To ensure that chair yoga remains a lifelong practice, it's important to approach it with both patience and enthusiasm. The following tips will help you build a sustainable, enjoyable routine that can accompany you through the years ahead:

1. **Start Small and Build Gradually**: Begin with short, manageable sessions, gradually increasing the time and complexity of your practice as you become more comfortable. This ensures that you don't overwhelm yourself and helps establish a habit that you can maintain in the long run.

2. **Stay Present**: One of the core aspects of chair yoga is

mindfulness. Stay present in each moment, focusing on your breath and how your body feels during each pose. This not only improves the effectiveness of the practice but also helps calm the mind and reduce stress.

3. **Celebrate Your Progress**: Recognize and celebrate the small victories—whether it's noticing less stiffness in your joints, holding a pose for longer, or feeling more relaxed after a session. Acknowledging these improvements can motivate you to keep going and reinforce the positive effects of your practice.

- 4. **Adjust as Needed**: As your body and lifestyle change, so should your practice. Don't be afraid to modify poses or try new techniques. If you encounter any challenges or physical limitations, consult a yoga instructor or healthcare provider for personalized modifications. Adaptability is key to maintaining a lifelong practice.

5. **Enjoy the Journey**: Above all, remember that chair yoga is not about perfection—it's about enjoying the process. Celebrate your journey, appreciate the present moment, and trust that the long-term benefits of chair yoga will unfold naturally as you

continue to invest in your health and wellness.

Chair yoga is a transformative practice that empowers seniors to live more vibrant, fulfilling lives. By embracing this gentle yet powerful form of movement, you'll cultivate physical strength, mental clarity, and emotional balance. Moving forward, remember that the key to a lifelong chair yoga practice is consistency, patience, and the willingness to listen to your body.

As you continue your journey, stay focused on the joy of movement and the health benefits that come with each breath and stretch. Let chair yoga be your companion for well-being, and allow it to support you

in navigating the challenges and joys
of aging with grace, vitality, and a
deep sense of peace.

Appendices

This section provides additional resources, definitions, and suggested reading to further enhance your chair yoga practice and overall well-being. Whether you're just beginning your journey or looking to deepen your knowledge, these appendices will serve as helpful tools in your ongoing exploration of chair yoga and mindfulness.

Chair Yoga Resources: Books, Apps, and Websites

Exploring additional resources can help enrich your chair yoga practice and provide valuable insights into yoga's broader benefits for seniors. Below are some recommended books, apps, and websites that you may find helpful:

Books:

1. "Chair Yoga: Sit, Stretch, and Strengthen Your Way to a Happier, Healthier You" by Kristi S. Shook
This accessible guide offers a variety of seated yoga poses and sequences that can be adapted for people of all abilities. It's a perfect book for seniors new to yoga or those looking to adapt their practice to a chair.

2. "Yoga for Healthy Aging: A Guide to Lifelong Well-Being" by Baxter Bell and Nina Zolotow
This book explores how yoga can help maintain flexibility, strength, and mental clarity as we age. It also offers

practices that can be tailored to your needs, with particular emphasis on joint health and balance.

3. "The Chair Yoga Bible: A Practical Guide to Seated Yoga for Seniors and Those with Limited Mobility" by Louise R. Sams

A comprehensive resource that offers step-by-step instructions for chair yoga poses, this book is specifically geared towards seniors and those with mobility limitations.

4. "Yoga and Arthritis: A Journey to Health and Healing" by Steffany Moonaz

For seniors dealing with arthritis, this book explains how yoga can help alleviate pain and improve mobility. It includes modifications and strategies for incorporating yoga into daily routines.

Apps:

1. **Daily Yoga**
This user-friendly app provides yoga sequences and instructional videos that cater to all experience levels, including beginner-friendly chair yoga routines.

2. **Yoga Studio by Gaiam**
Offering customizable yoga classes and sessions, this app allows you to select chair yoga practices based on your needs and preferences.

3. **Calm**

While not specifically for yoga, this app offers guided meditation, relaxation, and breathing exercises that complement a yoga practice and can help manage stress.

4. **MyYogaWorks**

With a variety of instructional videos and courses, MyYogaWorks features yoga routines designed for seniors, including those looking to practice yoga in a chair.

Websites:

1. **Yoga for Seniors (yogaforseniors.com)**

This website offers helpful guides, videos, and tips tailored specifically to seniors practicing yoga, including chair yoga techniques.

2. **Chair Yoga for Seniors (chairyogaforseniors.com)**

Dedicated to chair yoga, this site provides instructional resources, articles, and tips for seniors interested in adapting yoga to a seated position.

3. **Yoga Journal (yogajournal.com)**

A great resource for all things yoga, Yoga Journal offers articles, videos, and expert advice, including a section specifically on yoga for aging and mobility.

Glossary of Common Yoga Terms

Understanding common yoga terminology can help deepen your practice and make your journey smoother. Below are some key terms you may encounter during your chair yoga practice:

- **Asana**: The term for a specific yoga pose or posture.

- **Pranayama**: Breath control techniques used to calm and center the mind.

- **Vinyasa**: A style of yoga where movement flows with breath, typically faster-paced than chair yoga, but understanding this can help you appreciate the concept of breathwork.

- **Savasana**: A resting pose typically performed at the end of a yoga session, allowing the body to absorb the benefits of the practice.

- **Alignment**: The proper arrangement of your body during each pose to maximize safety and effectiveness.

- **Mindfulness**: The practice of being fully present and aware of your body, thoughts, and feelings during yoga.

- **Modifications**: Adjustments made to poses to suit individual needs, abilities, or limitations.

- **Chaturanga**: A yoga pose that involves lowering your body toward the floor, usually performed in standing yoga. It's helpful to understand as it's often referenced in videos or in teacher instructions.

Additional Mindfulness Practices for Seniors

While chair yoga offers a fantastic physical practice, mindfulness also plays a pivotal role in improving mental and emotional well-being. The following mindfulness practices can complement your chair yoga routine and enhance its benefits:

1. Deep Breathing Exercises:

Breathing deeply and slowly can trigger the body's relaxation response, lowering stress and anxiety. Practice taking deep, diaphragmatic breaths—inhale deeply through your nose, expanding your belly, and then exhale slowly through your mouth.

- **Practice**:
  Sit comfortably in your chair. Place one hand on your chest and the other on your abdomen. Inhale deeply through your nose, feeling your belly expand as it fills with air. Exhale slowly through your mouth. Repeat for 3-5 minutes.

2. Guided Meditation:

Meditation is a powerful tool for calming the mind, reducing stress, and improving mental clarity. Seniors can use short, guided meditation practices to relax before or after chair yoga sessions.

- **Practice**:
  Sit with a straight spine in your chair. Close your eyes and focus on your breath. Allow your thoughts to come and go without judgment. You can use a guided meditation app or simply focus on one calming word or phrase.

3. Body Scan Meditation:

This practice helps to develop body awareness and mindfulness. By mentally scanning each part of the body, seniors can identify areas of tension and release them.

- **Practice**:
  While seated, close your eyes and take a few deep breaths. Begin at your toes and mentally scan each part of your body, noticing any tension or discomfort. Consciously relax each area as you move upward, finishing with your head.

4. Loving-Kindness Meditation:

This type of meditation focuses on sending love and compassion to yourself and others. It's a wonderful practice for cultivating positive emotions and reducing stress.

- **Practice**:
  Sit comfortably and close your eyes. Begin by repeating to yourself: "May I be happy. May I be healthy. May I live with ease." Then, think of someone you care about and silently wish them the same.

Recommended Reading for Seniors

In addition to the specific resources for chair yoga, the following books and articles focus on topics like aging, mindfulness, and wellness that may complement your practice and offer deeper insights into living a fulfilling life as a senior:

1. "The Longevity Diet" by Valter Longo

This book focuses on how diet and lifestyle choices can promote longevity and improve health in aging.

2. "The Mindful Way Through Stress" by Shamash Alidina

An excellent resource for reducing stress through mindfulness and meditation practices, complementing the stress-relief benefits of yoga.

3. "The Art of Aging" by Sherwin B. Nuland

This book offers insights into the aging process, exploring how seniors can maintain mental and physical vitality.

4. "The Senior's Guide to Yoga" by Michael DeClemente

A practical guide to yoga for seniors, including advice on adapting poses for different abilities and needs.

5. "The Power of Now" by Eckhart Tolle

This spiritual classic helps readers live in the present moment, cultivating a mindset of peace and mindfulness, which is a key principle of yoga practice.

By exploring these resources and integrating additional mindfulness practices into your routine, you'll continue to enrich your chair yoga journey and embrace a fuller, healthier lifestyle. Each of these tools supports your overall well-being and enhances the lasting benefits of your chair yoga practice.